# WATER AEROBICS

# HOW TO LOSE WEIGHT AND TONE YOUR BODY IN THE WATER

## BY

## JENNIFER TAYLOR

*Health Warning*

If you are in any doubt as to your overall physical fitness then please consult your doctor before you perform any of the exercises contained within this book.

If you feel dizzy or exhausted whilst performing any of the routines in this book then please cease exercising immediately and consult a health professional.

# TABLE OF CONTENTS

## PLEASE REVIEW THIS BOOK

Thank you very much for buying this book. I hope you enjoy reading it as much as I have enjoyed writing it.

I would be very grateful if you would take the time to review this book on Amazon. I value all feedback.

Thank you so much!

Jennifer Taylor

Chapter 1 - Introduction

Do you want to burn fat without having to sweat? Or get toned without having to lift weights? Or even just return to normal health without the need for prescription medication?

If so, water aerobics is the PERFECT solution for you.

Walk or jump in the pool, burn some calories and have a whole lot of FUN.

You might break a sweat, but you won't know it. You will perform resistance training and cardio training exercises and you will ENJOY doing them.

You won't quit – why? The same reason why so many people keep doing Zumba every single week:

It's FUN and IT WORKS all at the same time!

So what is this book going to do for you?

It will help you:


*Discover all the BENEFITS of water aerobics...*

Like how you can improve strength, endurance, flexibility and cardiovascular health.

How you can decrease pain, risk of injury and impact on the joints.

How you can improve your posture, quality of sleep and life.

Or treat Parkinson's, Multiple Sclerosis and Rheumatoid Arthritis & More!

There are truly ENDLESS benefits to using water aerobics as your primary form of exercise.

### Find out what you need to KNOW, DO and EXPECT as a first-timer

For you, water aerobics is still new and that can be scary.

From preparing for your first visit, to warming up and completing the exercises properly, you will get to learn exactly what you need to know, do, and expect to be ready.

You don't need to feel embarrassed. Everybody has their own first time.

However, you CAN prepare yourself so that you are calm and confident.

### See the equipment and how to use it safely

One of the biggest fears in water aerobics comes from uncertainty.

Many are not sure how to perform the exercises.

The reality is that it comes down to knowing how to use the equipment.

If you know how all the equipment works, you're GOLD!

### View instructions & images on the BEST upper/lower body exercises

There are many water aerobic exercises, but some are better than others.

Find out which are the best and most popular and learn how to do them.

Equipped with illustrations of each exercise, this book will make sure you know:

1. How to perform the best UPPER body exercises;
2. How to perform the best LOWER body exercises; and
3. How to perform the best CARDIO exercises

So when you get in the water, there will be NO SURPRISES!

## *Learn how to CREATE YOUR OWN workout plan*

You get to learn all the fundamentals, then how to apply them.

Find out what is needed in a GOOD water aerobics workout program.

Create a plan of your own so you can work out with or without a class.

By the time you're done reading this book, you could even teach the class!

Chapter 2 – What Are The Benefits of Water Aerobics

Water aerobics is much more than just an effective way to get and stay in shape. It is a way to transform your entire health and lifestyle. It makes you feel better about yourself and the world around you. By training in water, you will gain the following types of health benefits: *body composition, cardiorespiratory, psychological, muscular system,* and *skeletal system*.

To address each of these benefits, let's first talk about the ones that make water aerobics better than many other forms of resistance, strength and cardio training.

1. **Water aerobics creates less impact on the joints.**

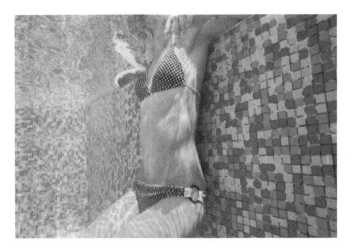

This is a big one, especially for women. Just picture yourself in water and think about how easy it is to jump. In fact, it's almost scary…you jump up without feeling limited by gravity, and if you don't know how to swim, well, you start to think about whether you will land before you actually do. That's beside the point, and the point is that water aerobics is less damaging to the joints.

What does this mean? It means that the rigorous pressure applied with typical strength, resistance and cardio training will not be a concern. The perfect example for this is running – it is absolutely horrible for your knees. Throw that out the window, get moving in the water and forget about the worry of hurting yourself.

No more knee problems, no more foot and leg injuries, no more back issues and for anyone with arthritis, simply NO MORE PAIN!

This is not just in theory; the truth is that being submerged in water will cause your body weight to decrease. This can happen to the extent of 50-90% of your non-soaked body weight, depending on the level of the water. This puts a lot less resistance to the same movements you would perform out of the water, which means significantly less pressure on the joints.

Further, water aerobics exercises are created with joint impact in mind. This is accomplished by requiring the exerciser to limit range of motion to 60-70% of the movement. In return, this will prevent hyperextension of the joints and allow for maximum protection of the joints while working out.

2. **Safe exercise option for those affected by medical conditions.**

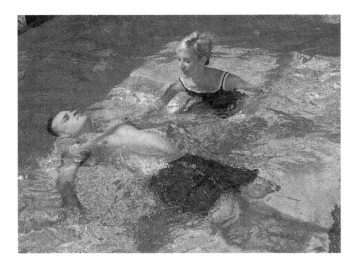

One of the worst things about falling ill to any disorder, disease, or whatever it may be, is that it tends to send your life into a downward spiral. You begin to have your life controlled by the condition. You may have difficulty with even the simplest weight training and cardio exercises, your work productivity may be hindered, and chasing around a little one, well you may as well forget it.

You know who you are – this either speaks to you or it doesn't.

You may suffer from Parkinson's, Multiple Sclerosis, Rheumatoid Arthritis, Osteoporosis, Fibromyalgia, or even obesity, but it doesn't matter!

All these conditions can only restrict you so much. Once you get into water, you can literally feel weight being lifted off your shoulder. You are no longer held back by your medical problems. You can exercise and start to feel healthy and fit again.

And you know what?

If you make a routine out of water aerobics, you can start to see recovery from the painful symptoms associated with any of these conditions. You can start to feel more comfortable getting out of bed each day. You can start to take control of your life again!

That is not to say that there will not be challenges along the way. If you are someone that deals with any physically-damaging condition then there will be some limitations that you will have. This is why it is sometimes better to stick with small classes so you have an instructor available that has dealt with special conditions such as yours. If you are very concerned then you could even seek a physical therapist that offers in-water physical therapy.

It will only take 20 minutes of your time, maybe four days a week, and you will really start to notice relief from your pain symptoms.

### 3. Lose weight without sweating or injuring yourself.

The weight loss aspect of water aerobics is mostly focused around two key components, which are as follows: the *lack of physical exertion required to succeed*, and, the *reduced risk of injury*.

Think about jumping in water again. You jump up with ease. Now think about the process of jumping outside of water. Not nearly as easy is it? If you have a medical condition that hinders your physical ability, then jumping outside of water may even be impossible.

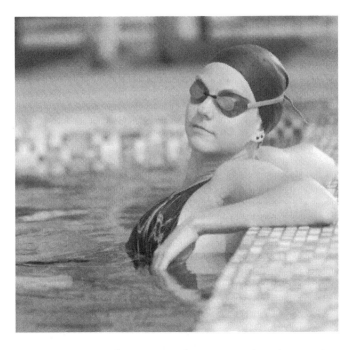

Thankfully, the buoyancy of water makes it so that EVERYONE can exercise and see results. In a matter of only a few weeks you will start to feel and look slimmer. Not only that, but by hopping on a set of scales you will find out that you ARE thinner!

Yes, weight loss is not a magical process. You will have to look at your diet too. But, water aerobics makes for an extremely easy and fun way to burn calories.

### How many calories can you burn in water?

Well, that all depends on your physical exertion level, body weight and metabolism.

According to *Mayo Clinic*, one hour of exercise will burn approximately:

- 402 calories for someone 160 pounds (73kg)
- 501 calories for someone 200 pounds (91kg)
- 600 calories for someone 240 pounds (109kg)

If weight loss is your main goal, and you treat water aerobics as your primary exercise and put all your energy into it, then you could easily burn even more than the stated amounts.

To put it into perspective, assume you burn 500 calories per hour and perform water aerobics for four hours per week. This equates to 2,000 calories burnt every single week. That's over 8,000 calories in a month. Guess what? It only takes a 3,500 caloric deficit to lose one pound – and we haven't even touched the caloric intake from your diet!

So you could easily find yourself losing well over two extra pounds per month, just by performing water aerobics four times a week. Not too shabby for such a fun and easy form of exercise.

### 4. Improve strength, resistance, and endurance.

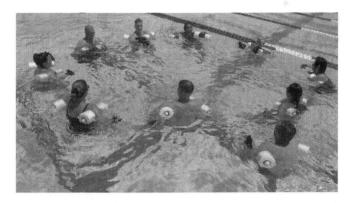

Water aerobics isn't just for building a smaller person, it's for building a BETTER person.

By sticking to a routine, you will be able to achieve considerable strength and endurance improvements. All this will make you feel stronger and healthier every single day.

Firstly, let's look at the strength improvements.

Muscular strength is improved due to applied force fighting resistance. Think about jumping with ankle weights. The weight tries to weigh you down, but while you're jumping FORCE fights the resistance of these weights. The same can be applied in the water. When making any movement, which obviously requires the application of force, the water will serve as a resistance.

There is no doubt that water alone would not be sufficient to overload the muscles, or at least not for long. Muscular strength training is new for many. If that's the case for you, then you will easily notice some strength improvements at first. However, it won't take long before you will need to start using water aerobics equipment to continue seeing these improvements.

Then, you have the endurance improvements.

Endurance is built from repetition and duration. If you stick to the water aerobics workout program and remain consistent, then you will notice some endurance improvements. These will become much more noticeable if your program is centered on high repetition movements. It is these movements that are also best for weight loss purposes.

Think about it this way:
When you lift weights, you increase strength by adding resistance and fighting more force into the movement. The same applies with your endurance, but in different context.

Endurance is dictated by how long you can last given the particular movement. Therefore, your endurance can be improved by continuously doing more repetitions or working out for longer periods of time.

If you have very low endurance, then it may be a good idea to build this up before working on your strength. For anyone that is obese, this may also be a good option since endurance training will trigger weight loss and you will likely want to lose weight before adding many strength movements into your program.

### 5. Improve your posture, quality of sleep and mood.

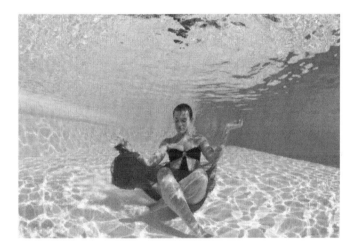

With or without a medical illness, poor posture remains common. It may be due to naturally slanting your body growing up. It may also be because of weak back muscles. Or, it could be a result of a medical condition.

Regardless of why you have bad posture, you *can* improve it by strengthening your skeletal structure. The change won't happen overnight, but by spending months in and out remaining physically active, you will definitely start to notice a difference.

The same goes for your quality of sleep. Whether you have any sleeping disorders, or you just have difficulty getting to sleep on time, staying asleep all night, etc., you will be able to see some benefit from being consistent with your water aerobics training.

Why is this? Aside from the relaxation that being in water gives your body, you are getting physically active and giving yourself a reason to be tired. This is especially true for many that suffer from a physically-hindering medical condition, because they do not get active and go through their day being mostly sedentary.

Exercising regularly allows for sufficient levels of serotonin to be released within the brain. This is the chemical that is responsible for assisting you in getting a good night's sleep. It is also the chemical that, when released, makes you feel HAPPY.

By getting physically active, and doing it within a routine, you will certainly start to notice that you can get to sleep easier and you will also notice that your body will be rested and well-rejuvenated the next day. With time, you may even notice that your posture is beginning to improve. Further, you or the people around you will start to notice that you are actually happier and have a more positive balance of moods.

Aside from these major benefits, there are still many more great improvements that often go unnoticed. This includes the following:

- Improved flexibility of the muscles;
- Decreased amount of muscle mass loss;

- Increased level of muscle maintenance;
- Enhanced range of motion of muscles and joints;
- Slowed degeneration of joints;
- Reduced level of memory loss;
- Bettered physical image and sexual appeal;
- Inhibited metabolism decrease from aging;
- Controlled or normalized blood pressure levels; and
- Heightened efficiency of the heart.

Chapter 3 – What Every Beginner Should Know

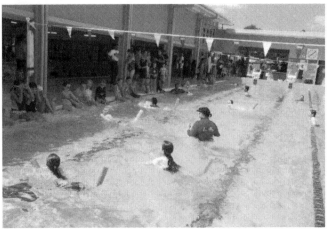

*Photo by Brisbane City Council*

Now that we have covered many of the amazing benefits that water aerobics has to offer, it is important to begin looking at what you need to know BEFORE you jump in the pool.

Water aerobics is easy enough to get into if you join a class and attend from the very first day, but it is not always a case of black and white. Whether you are jumping mid-way into a course or you are planning to exercise on your own, there are quite a few things that you will want to know so you are comfortable and confident when you finally get started.

What you need to know breaks down into safety, equipment and exercises. The safety factors are very important as you want to make sure that you are not putting yourself at risk by performing these exercises. The equipment is relatively basic and easy to use, but knowing how it all works ahead of time is always good. The exercises are something that requires a bit more attention, which is why they will be covered in the following chapters.

**SAFETY**

Water aerobics does not consist of any truly dangerous exercises. However, since many choose this type of exercise for its low impact and compatibility with various physical conditions, it is important to make sure you know your level of ability before beginning. It is also essential to confirm that it will be safe for you to start exercising in the water at this time.

What should you do? It's simple – consult with your doctor before starting water aerobics!

This is not necessary if you deem yourself as completely healthy and in good shape. However, it may be important to speak with your physician prior to performing water aerobics if you suffer from any medical condition that may hinder your athletic performance and ability, or that may be worsened as a result of physical exercise.

Further, breathing is an important part of all aerobics exercises, and this should be treated no differently when performing them in water. Breathing isn't difficult at all, but you need to know how to breathe properly so that you can safely and effectively perform any water aerobics exercise.

## Proper Breathing Techniques

The importance of breathing falls under the necessity of providing oxygen to fatigued muscles. This provides you with further endurance and will limit the risk of injury. It is something that is often overlooked, but in the bodybuilding and powerlifting worlds, it can be noticed as key components of exercise.

The key to providing oxygen to your muscles is **deep breathing** – this is easier said than done though, as many do not know how to properly perform a deep breath.

Here is a step-by-step guide that will teach you how to breathe properly when performing water aerobics exercises:

1. Breathe in (through your NOSE)
2. Push stomach out (as breathing in)
3. Breathe out (through your MOUTH)
4. Let stomach in (as breathing out)

It really is that simple and the only difference for most people is that you will be breathing through your stomach instead of through your chest. Try it out a few times right now and you will notice that it feels both smooth and natural to breathe this way.

## Types of Equipment

First off, there will be no getting around the need for a swimming pool. While, in theory, you could complete these workouts at a beach, it's definitely not the way to go. So, assuming you have a swimming pool or access to one, you will then want to look at equipment that can enhance your workout experience.

The equipment that you can get or use will usually do one of two things – increase resistance or improve balance.

As there are many different pieces of equipment that could be used, this section will cover them all. Images will be provided to display what each piece of equipment looks like. You will be able to obtain these items from www.amazon.com, www.ebay.com or a specialist water aerobics website like www.water-aerobics-shop.com.

Here it goes…

1) Balls (preferably 10" in diameter)

**Uses:** Many water aerobics exercises include beach balls, typically 10 inches in diameter. Different sizes may be used for certain exercises and may provide different balance and resistance effects. Typically, balls are used in water aerobics for movements like the Ball Lever, the Single Leg Ball Extension and Aquatic Basketball. A ball may be thrown into many different exercises and a bit of trial and error may be used to see which exercises it can be used to provide additional support or resistance.

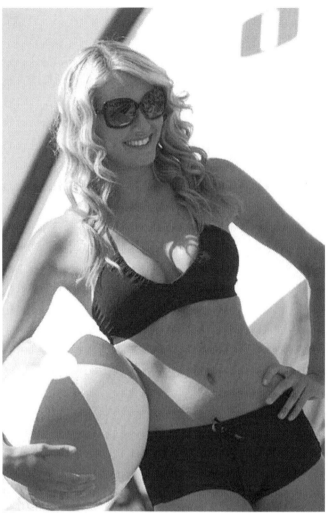

*Photo by Magnus Manske*

2) Hand Buoys

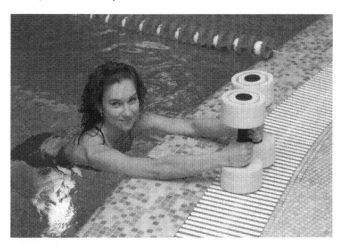

**Uses:** The hand buoy is a type of specialty water weight that adds resistance to water aerobics movements, especially those that target the upper body. These specialty hand weights are made in varying types of materials, which may play into the overall resistance increase that they create. The product in the image is the Hydro-Fit Hand Buoy. These particular hand buoys are made out of closed cell Ethafoam, which is a very high quality and water-friendly material. While designs vary, this particular product is made with emphasis on decreasing tension to the shoulders and wrists. They can also be found in Regular, Jumbo and Mini size – the difference in size affects the resistance and buoyancy that the buoys will create when in use.

This piece of equipment is fairly important in a water aerobics workout as it is needed for a large number of exercises. This includes movements such as the Bicep Curls, Rows, and Cross Country Ski.

3)  Pool Noodles

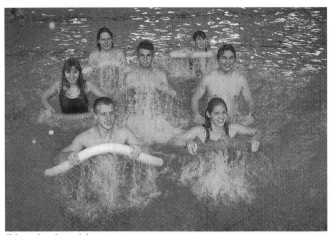

*Photo by: http://www.royan.com.ar*

**Uses:** The pool noodle is one of the most common pieces of equipment in a water aerobics workout. This is because it is so versatile and comes into play for both resistance and balance support purposes. The pool noodle can be found in countless exercises, such as the Stair Master, the Backward Leg Raise, the Mermaid Moment, the Hip Abduction & Adduction, and the Noodle Leg Extensions.

4)  Kickboards

**Uses:** The kickboard is a valuable tool for a water aerobics workout because it helps with improving balance while both sitting and standing and it can be used to enhance resistance during waist movements. While the Centerfold is the only exercise in this guide that uses kickboards, there are still many different exercises that may require this particular piece of equipment. It can also be used as you wish to improve balance during certain other movements.

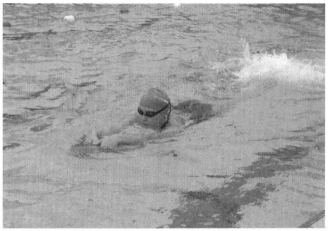

*Photo by www.simplyswim.com*

5)  Stabilization Bar

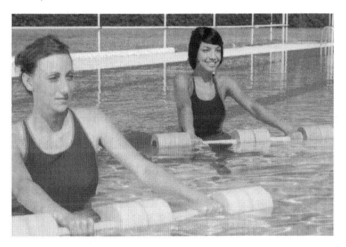

**Uses:** The stabilization bar does not necessarily add options of exercises to a water aerobics workout. However, for those that have stability or balance issues, it can definitely add to the amount of exercises that you will be able to do on your own. The reason for this is simple – the stabilization bar creates the stability that you need in order to be able to effectively perform various exercises. Sometimes, a pool noodle will not be effective enough to ensure that you keep balance and for safety and performance purposes, this may serve as a better alternative. An example of an exercise that this may be true for is the Backward Leg Raise, which requires a considerable amount of balance to perform.

When purchasing a stabilization bar, the main consideration will be the length. From the image example, this particular stabilization bar model is available in both three and four foot designs. The cost is slightly higher for the longer bar.

6)  Aquatic Gloves

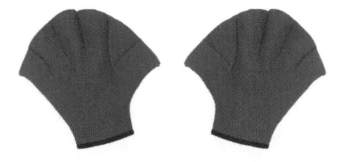

**Uses:** While the aquatic gloves are not an essential item to own for a water aerobics workout, they still have a lot to offer. These gloves are perfect for the Karate Punch and Aquatic Kickboxing exercises found in this guide and they are useful for any other striking and punching styled movements as well. Basically, aquatic gloves will increase the intensity of quick arm movements. While most users choose aquatic gloves for performance reasons, some will also decide that they are worth buying as they can protect the fingers from cold pool water, which can otherwise cause the hands to go numb.

7) Resistance Bands

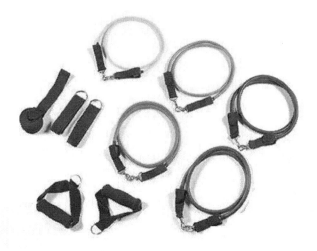

*Photo by: www.trenirai.me*

**Uses:** There are countless potential exercises that can be performed with resistance bands. While a basic resistance band would suffice for most purposes, there are more advanced systems available as well. The image provided is of a resistance band system near the higher end of the retail price range. The idea of this large, multi-item system is that it can be used in place of many other resistance devices. In this particular example, you have resistance bands with hand and leg attachments, an inflatable belt featuring back support, standard resistance bands, high pressure suction cups, and more.

Resistance bands are used in many different movements. Chest flies is the only particular movement found in this guide that actually uses resistance bands. However, it can be used in place of other items to add resistance to other movements, such as the Bicep Curl and the Shoulder Shrug.

8) Ankle Weights

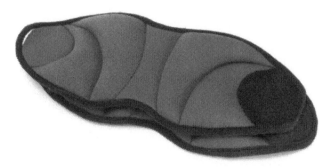

**Uses:** Ankle weights are designed to provide an increased level of resistance while performing lower body exercises. Some examples of movements in this guide that can be increased in difficulty with ankle weights include the Forward Leg Raise, the Backward Leg Raise, the Single Leg Raise and the Single Leg Ball Extension. Ankle weights are available in various weight amounts; the image displays ankle weights that are five pounds on each side. The cost of these weights may vary according to the actual weight.

9) Hand Weights

**Uses:** Hand weights are designed to provide an increased level of resistance while performing exercises that requires movement of the arms. Some examples of movements in this guide that can be increased in difficulty with hand weights include the Karate Punch, Rows, Shoulder Shrugs and Aquatic Kickboxing.

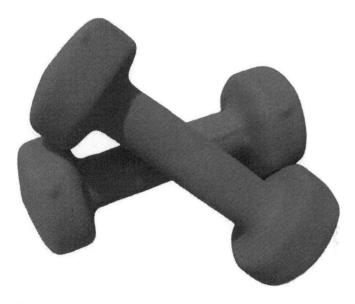

*Photo by Aasimovic*

Hand weights can be found in different weight amounts; the image is of hand weights that are five pounds each. The cost may vary slightly depending on the weight, but mostly varies by brand and store. This particular design is appealing as it offers wrist support and lowers tension on the joints as a result of additional weight in the movement.

Chapter 4 – Warming up & Cooling Down

## *Warm up*

As with any type of exercise, for safety and overall performance ability purposes, it is essential that you make sure to both warm up and cool down before and after performing water aerobics exercises.

For water aerobics, the warm up process is essential to get blood and oxygen flowing, to get the heart rate up and to get the joints stretched out.

There are many different warm up exercises that you can perform. Here is an example of an effective method to warm up before performing water aerobics exercises:

Perform a brisk walk or march in place for between five and eight minutes while in the shallow end of the pool. Gradually include different types of arm movements while you march or walk. This may include putting your arms ahead of you, behind you, crossing them, etc.

As you notice an increase in heart rate, you can transition into performing jumping jacks. This will allow you to further get your heart rate up and will get you into a more intense training zone.

Now, you should switch to a high-heeled jog. When you have done this for long enough, you may finish up your warm up with ankle touches to the front and heel touches to the back.

That's it!

Also, there is no set amount of time that you really have to do any of the movements or motions for as all you really need to achieve is the following three things:

1)  An increase in heart rate;
2)  An increase in body temperature; and
3)  An increase in flexibility of the joints.

Elevating your heart rate will make it easier to perform more intensive exercises without having issues as a result of a sudden spike in heart rate. Elevating your body temperature will allow your body to lower the risk of overheating and dehydration. Enhancing flexibility of the joints will decrease the risk of injury when performing more physically demanding exercises.

If this warm up example is not for you, another option is to perform a short jog in place, switch to multiple scissor kicks, perform wide sweeping movements with the arms, and continuing with the flow for a few minutes before beginning your lighter exercises.

## Cool down

The cool down process is just as important as the warm up phase. After you are done the heart of your workout, your muscles and joints will have gotten worked up and need to be relaxed in order to prevent injury. This can require as much as 20 minutes of cool down exercise which may consist of a routine that is very similar to the warm up process.

When performing the cool down routine, the main focus will be in cooling down the particular muscles and joints that have been worked throughout the workout.    These will be targeted through various fluid movements and with a gradual decrease in intensity.

For example, you may return to performing wide sweeping movements with the arms, scissor kicks, jog in place, and then end the workout with a brisk walk or by marching for a few minutes.

In the end, you will be bringing your heart rate back down, as you would with a cool down phase for any other type of exercise. For example, running on the treadmill is typically done by gradually increasing the speed and then cooling down by gradually returning to a walking speed. This is very important as the major heart rate spikes that would be experienced without a warm up or cool down before and after your water aerobics workout can be very dangerous to your health and can increase the risk of injury.

In this next section, details and instructions will be provided on certain movements that can be performed during the warm up and cool down stages of your water aerobics routine. This will include a basic description of each of these exercises, which will be followed by a detailed guide on how to perform them.

## EXERCISES

### Thermal Warm Up

**What it is:** Thermal warm up consists of light movements that work to get the body temperature up. This allows for an increased level of oxygen to the muscles during the workout. It also assists with synovial fluid release from the joints. This part of the warm up will begin with short, then transition to long lever exercises. It can be performed at various intensity levels, which means that it may be done by anyone regardless of their current fitness and flexibility levels.

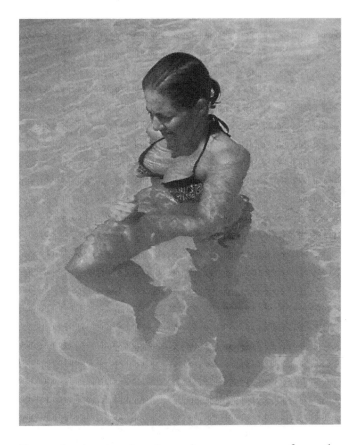

**Example:** jogging in place. As you can see from the image, the motion is limited and creating an L-shaped range of motion, which creates a short lever. This only requires a bit of force and is low in intensity.

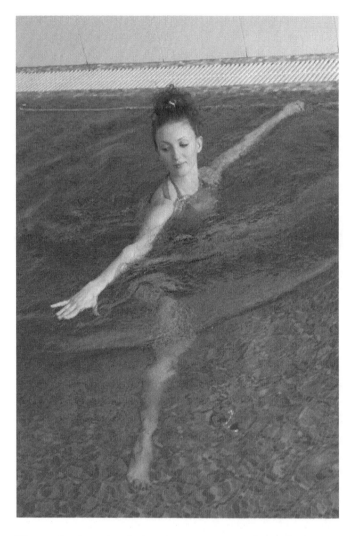

**Example:** jumping jacks. As you can see from the image, nearly the entire leg is brought into the movement. This creates a larger range of motion and a longer lever. It requires a bit more force than the short lever example and requires a higher level of intensity, but is still not too restricting based on one's fitness levels as the movement can still be performed to some extent.

**Toy Soldier March**

**What it is:** Imagine a toy soldier, simply marching in place. That is exactly what you need to do for this exercise. Simple enough, right? You can make it a little tougher by speeding up the movements. This is by far one of the easiest warm up exercises to perform. In slower execution, absolutely everyone will be able to perform the exercise without any real issue. You can choose whether to speed it up and how fast to speed it up to if you wish to pick up the pace at any point, so your physical shape will not interfere with your ability to perform the exercise.

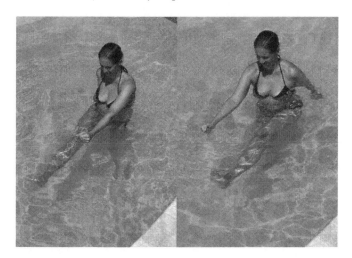

**What to do:** with a relaxed jaw and shoulders, and firm posture, as well as loosened hands and elbows, simply lift knees in every step and lift the opposing hand to the height of your chest. Continue doing this as if you are marching alongside an actual marching band, but don't waste too much energy – it's a warm up!

## Can Can Kick

**What it is:** From marching band to showgirls, the Can Can Kick originated from the idea of kicking a can and made its way to sensual stage dancing. In a more conservative manner, the Can Can Kick also works as a good long lever warm up exercise. It is a bit more difficult to perform for someone with a restricted level of flexibility in the legs, but a similar range of motion for the same movement can be performed with the same results.

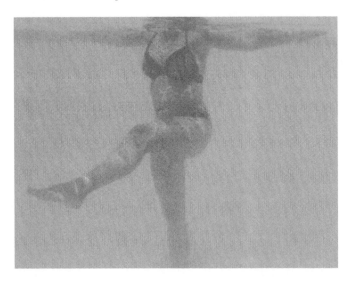

**What to do:** with firm posture and balanced arms, and while standing on the "tippy-toes" of your opposite leg, simply 'kick a can' by performing a high kick. Ideally, you will create an L-shape with your legs, but kicking as high as you comfortably can is fine.

## Side Knee Hop

**What it is:** The side knee hop looks like jogging or running in place while in water, but it is actually a jumping exercise. It is also very easy to perform and due to the low impact nature of doing it within the water, there should be no issues for anyone attempting this particular warm up exercise. It is one of the more basic short lever exercises that you can perform.

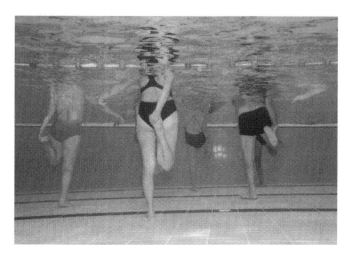

**What to do:** with one leg restricted, the other firmly planted down, and a tall posture, simply perform a one legged jump. The restriction to the non-jumping leg may be accomplished either by holding it back as in the picture, or by simply leaning it forward or backward. To add a bit of balancing challenge to the exercise, you can create an L-shape by either lifting the opposing leg completely forward or as far back as possible prior to performing the jump.

**Treading Water**

**What it is:** Treading water is the process of using your arms and/or legs to keep your head above water. This is a technique that it used while remaining stagnant in deep water, whether in a swimming pool or out in the ocean. You can tread water while staying in place, and partially while moving in any direction as well. This is considered as one of the more boring warm ups and is often not labelled as an exercise of its own, but it is something that will be performed regularly if you are not keeping in the shallow end of the pool while performing your water aerobics routine.

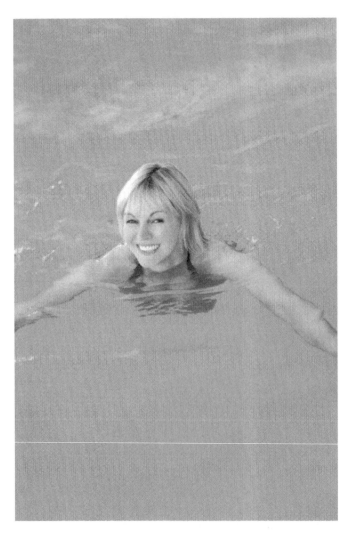

**What to do:** keep your head above water by kicking your arms or legs repetitively, almost in the manner of performing the "doggy paddle" swimming technique. This is a technique that you will likely already know, but you will want to make sure that you completely understand the process if you have not done it before.

**Wave Makers**

**What it is:** The wave maker is a move that is done essentially with the effort of creating waves within the pool. It is done in the most aggressive way possible to achieve these results, which happens to be through an exercise that not only works core strength, but the abdominal, leg, butt and back muscles as well. It is also relatively easy for just about everyone to complete and can be done at varying levels of intensity.

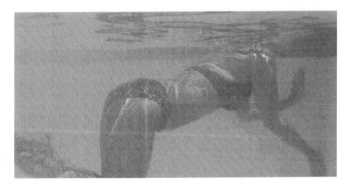

**What to do:** head deep enough into the pool so that you are submerged to around chest level in the water. While facing in the direction of the pool edge, use your left hand to hold onto the edge of the pool. Then, place the palm of your right hand onto the pool wall while the hand is submerged in water. This is then followed by creating an extension to the legs, positioned directly behind you, with your knees and feet stuck together. Then, begin performing a flapping motion with your legs, almost like a dolphin's tail.

Typically, you will want to perform the flapping motion for roughly 30 seconds, creating heavy waves that come above the water surface. You can decrease your speed and perform basic flutter kicks with your legs spread apart if you begin to run out of energy.

## Water Kicks

**What it is:** Water kicks are simply kicks that are done while your legs are submerged in water, but there are a few variations to them that can be performed. The major difference between styles of water kicking for warm up and cool down purposes is the direction in which the kick is made. Regardless, the movements are typically all long lever exercises and can be performed at varying levels of intensity.

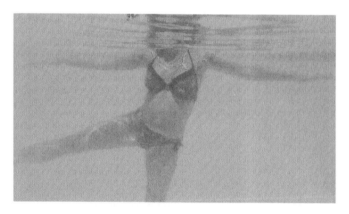

**What to do:** With a tall posture, loose arms and strong balance, simply perform a leg kick in any direction. This may be done frontward, sideways or backward. In the image example, the individual is performing a side kick as the leg is being lifted towards the side. This move is also performed with some level of force, but the extent of intensity is completely up to you and lower intensity kicks may be performed to warm up and cool down

- Stretching is recommended after your cool down period. Here are some quick suggestions:

*Calves*

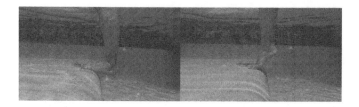

You can stretch your calf muscles out by heading to the pool stairs, stepping onto the edge of a step, and let your heel hang off of the step while standing on your toes. From here, begin to gradually lower your body down until you have accomplished a full stretch in the calf muscles. You should repeat this movement nine more times, for a total of 10 repetitions. Make sure that you do not try to force the stretch as the natural movement is what matters.

*Legs*

You can stretch your leg muscles out by lifting your leg onto the side of the pool (at a depth that is comfortable to you), and carefully lowering your head down. You can switch it up by going as far down with your head on one leg, and then the other. Also, be sure that you are slowly moving into the stretch and not bouncing yourself as doing so could lead to injury.

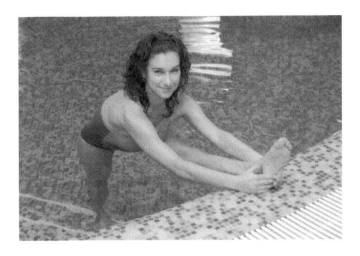

*Shoulders*

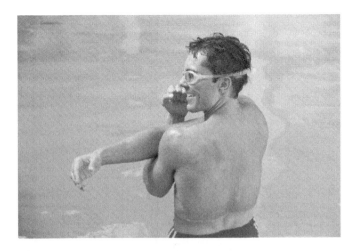

You can stretch your shoulder muscles in a number of ways. The first way would be to hold your hand on a door frame with your arm lifted up and bend your arm back by leaning forward. This may not be easily done when just getting out of a pool. Another way is to position your hands like a prayer behind your back and move them up towards your neck as much as you comfortably can, but make sure this is done slowly and carefully. The last option would be to lift one arm up with a bend in the elbow near your head and your hand running down to your back and cross your other arm above your head and hold onto the elbow. The shoulder stretch is very important as it will contribute towards loosening the upper arms and back, which often get type from water aerobics, especially when you have worked out with hand weights. The shoulder stretch will also stretch your triceps.

**NOTE:** These are only some of the basic stretches that you can do after a water aerobics workout. It is important that you figure out a stretching routine that works for your body. You can look further into the different options of static stretches and other types of stretches by muscle group by visiting the EXRX - Stretching page.

Chapter 5 – Upper Body Workout

Water aerobics is a full body workout. It is broken down into many exercises which target all areas of the body. The warm up and cool down exercises simply serve as a way to get the entire body ready for the workout. Once you get into your workout you will be performing a variety of exercises and hitting all of the body's muscle groups.

While some movements can work multiple muscle groups at the same time, many other exercises target a particular part of the body. In general, it is easiest to classify exercises within the workout as either: Upper Body; Lower Body; or Cardio.

This chapter will cover the UPPER BODY workout. This consists of all water aerobics exercises that specifically target the upper portion of the body. This would be any exercises that hit muscles above the waist line.

Interestingly enough, many of the upper body exercises are comparable to weight lifting exercises that target the upper portion of the body. This includes some of the more common exercises, such as Bicep Curls, Chest Flies, Shoulder Shrugs and Rows.

To make it easier, let's just jump right in to 10 examples of highly effective upper body water aerobics exercises.

  1)   Bicep Curls

**What it is:** Bicep curls feature a very basic movement that targets the bicep brachii, which is the muscle found in the top side of the upper arm. This isolated exercise is very basic, but it works great with resistance training and provides a good mix of resistance and intensity when performed as a water aerobics exercise.

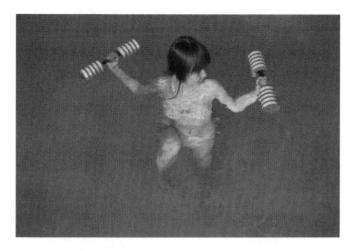

**What to do:** As you can see in the picture, your hands will be placed with a supinated grip (think: holding a bowl of soup), which places the palms facing up. The individual creates a firm, yet relaxed grip on the dumbbell, water bottle or whatever piece of equipment is used.

The movement will begin with the weighted equipment held slightly above the chest. The arms will have a natural slight inward position. The movement begins with the lowering of the weight and the motion is then reversed after the weight reaches close to your thighs. This must be done as a controlled movement and the elbows must be kept close to the body for the whole range of motion.

**Equipment Needed:** To perform a bicep curl in water, you simply need something that can be held and moved with the needed range of motion. In many water aerobics classes, a water bottle full of water is commonly used for this exercise. Alternatively, you may use other pieces of water aerobics equipment for this exercise, such as a lightweight dumbbell and specialty water weights.

2)  Chest Flies

**What it is:** Chest flies are a type of isolated chest exercise that crosses over from the bodybuilding world. This particular exercise is perfect for resistance training purposes and serves well if done properly when in water. However, given the nature of the movement, it can be difficult to perform if you do not have the right equipment.

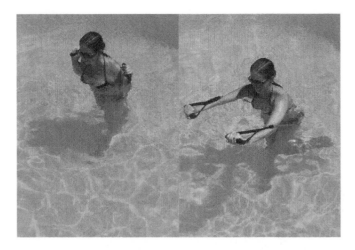

**What to do:** In this image, you can see an individual standing in chest-height water levels with a resistance band stabilized by her back foot. The handles of the resistance band are held comfortably around the shoulders and chest, with the hands gripping and positioned as if throwing a punch.

The hands are moved to near full extension, ending just short of where the elbows would lock out. At this point, you will want to squeeze and create tension within the chest muscles. On the reverse of the motion, there will be resistance forced in to increase the intensity of the exercise. Depending on the height level at which the exercise is performed, it is possible to target the lower, upper or middle of the chest, but in general, it remains as an overall chest exercise.

**Equipment Needed:** This exercise is demonstrated with a resistance band, which is the perfect piece of equipment as it naturally enforces the tension that is necessary to make this particular exercise work as best as it can.

3)   Shoulder Shrugs

**What it is:** The shoulder shrug is an exercise that targets the upper trapezius muscles in the back of the shoulders. This particular exercise is the most common choice for anyone weightlifting with the intention of growing large trap muscles or big shoulders overall. However, it is also commonly used in water aerobics workouts as it is an effective resistance training exercise for the shoulder muscles.

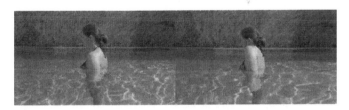

**What to do:** As you can see, the movement begins with the weights grasped in hammer grip fashion, which consists of a firm grasp on the weights and the palm facing in towards the body.

With both arms strictly in place, the weights are moved directly upward. This brings the shoulders inward towards the neck a bit when the top of the movement is reached.

There is a squeeze and creation of tension in the shoulders at the top of the movement. The weight is then cautiously lowered back to the starting position.

**Equipment Needed:** This exercise is performed simply with weight that can be held in the hands while in water. Due to the increased resistance from the water, only a very lightweight dumbbell would be necessary. Alternatively, you can also perform this exercise with specialty water weights. A resistance band would not be as good as it would be more difficult to complete the straight up and down range of motion without any directional interference.

4)  Rows

**What it is:** Rows are one of the most common upper body exercises in existence. They are a very straightforward exercise, which are designed to target the back muscles. Depending on the hand positioning and movement direction, they may target the middle or upper back. The latissimus dorsi muscles, which are the large back muscles on the back, in line with the chest muscles, are often targeted in an isolated movement, but the trapezius, rhomboid, and deltoid muscles are all commonly hit as well.

**What to do:** The picture below should give you an idea on how your hands should be placed. In this example, the individual is positioned so that her arms are at the top of the water, which allows for the weight to move while still submerged in the water. This is important as you want to keep the water-induced resistance in place.

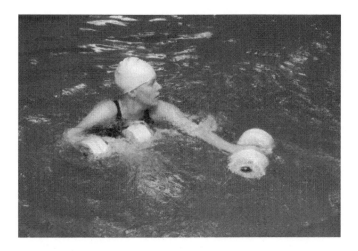

The movement begins with the weight held in almost full extension, positioned with the arm directly in front of the individual. In this example, an overhanded grip is used to perform the movement. The motion begins by drawing the arm back, while keeping the same overall positioning. There will be a slight squeeze in the targeted back muscle at the end of the motion, which occurs when the elbow has just breached parallel level with the body. The reverse of the movement is performed with slight resistance and the exercise is reset when the elbows have almost locked out.

**Equipment Needed:** This movement is most commonly performed with either a lightweight dumbbell or specialty water weights. Some will choose to use water bottles full of water as a quick fix for a lack of water aerobics equipment. Resistance bands can also be used, but it is difficult for this exercise as they will need to be attached to something at the appropriate height level in order for them to work properly for this movement.

5) Karate Punch

**What it is:** Simple enough, the karate punch is nothing more than the punch that is used when practicing karate. With this punch, the intention is to make contact with the first two knuckles of the hand – the index and middle finger knuckles. The only point that should be made is that any involvement of other parts of the hand will ultimately classify the movement as a karate strike instead of a karate punch. Also, there are no worries if this seems like something that is too difficult as you do not need to have perfect form in order to get the benefits from it in a water aerobics workout.

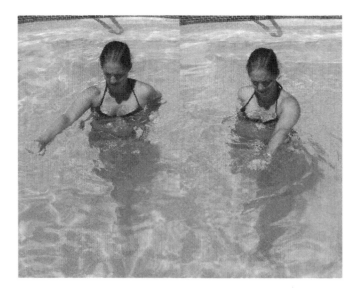

**What to do:** You can see from the picture above that the individual is exercising specifically with a punching motion.

To perform a karate punch in water, you simply need to create a straight line for the punching motion and make sure to turn your hand over at the very last second of the movement. Make sure to create a straight line punch – punching straight in and straight out.

**Equipment Needed:** This exercise can be performed without any equipment as it is merely a punching movement. However, it is possible to use punching gloves and mitts for this exercise as well. You can also use a water bottle full of water, specialty water weights, or a lightweight dumbbell to effectively perform the karate punch while in water.

6) Ball Lever

**What it is:** This innovative water aerobics exercise allows you to essentially turn yourself into a lever for the ball that is used for the movement. The idea is that you are controllably moving the ball from one height to another. Typically, the ball will be moved from in front of you to around your thigh area.

**What to do:** While grabbing onto the ball, hold it in front of you with your arms stretched out as much as possible. During this time, you will be floating in chest-high water with your face positioned downward. Your legs will be extended back as far as possible and your feet will be kept together. With the arms positioned straight ahead, drag the ball underneath you and with all your force, pull it as quickly as possible toward the thighs. After it reaches this location, create a bend in the elbows and press the ball ahead to retract to the starting position for the movement.

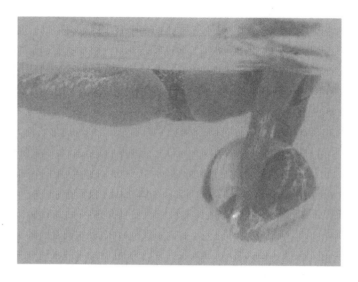

At the beginner level, it is acceptable to keep your head above water while completing this exercise. To make it a little more difficult, you can perform it with your head under water. If you choose this method, it is important to remember to take advantage of your chance to breathe during the movement. This will be possible while the ball is below you as it will cause you to lift above the water and you will have time to take a quick breathe before going back under.

**Equipment Needed:** The only equipment that is necessary for this particular exercise is a ball. Typically, a small beach ball will suffice for this movement. To make the exercise more difficult, you can switch a small beach ball out for a larger one. Regardless, to maximize muscle sculpting benefits, it is essential to keep focus on strictly straight limbs during the movement before worrying about increasing difficulty with different equipment.

7)    Single Leg Ball Extension

**What it is:** The single leg ball extension is an exercise that works to effectively strengthen the abdominal and shoulder muscles. It also helps with building balance and slightly improves strength in the legs. It is a straightforward exercise and is performed as a controlled movement.

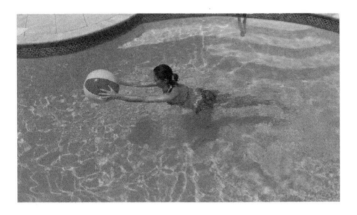

**What to do:** As you can see in the picture, you are essentially creating a balance with your leg while holding a ball out in front of you. This movement begins with only the ball positioned directly in front of the individual. At this point, either one of the legs can be extended back with the toes pointed back. The abdomen is kept tight through the entire movement.

To start the movement, draw the ball down towards your waist area. Do this while maintaining a slight bend in the elbows and retract the legs towards the center. Continue performing this movement while switching between legs after each repetition.

**Equipment Needed:** This exercise only requires the individual to have a ball. A beach ball will usually suffice for this particular movement. The difficulty can be increased slightly by simply using a larger beach ball. This should be avoided until you have mastered the exercise and you have determined that there are no issues with balancing throughout the entire movement.

8)  Centerfold

**What it is:** This is a core exercise that targets the abdominal muscles. This is one of the more complex movements as it requires a transition between positions in order to achieve the full range of motion. However, it is not too difficult to complete and it is highly effective at targeting your abs.

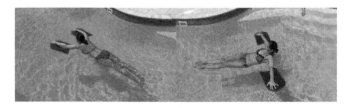

**What to do:** With your arms placed on kickboards directly in front of you, float above the water while facing downward and your legs positioned back with your toes pointed. Create a bend in your knees and begin to bring your legs underneath you. At the same time, draw your arms in and create a 90 degree angle. This will bring you to an upright position. From here, take your time and transition to having your legs straight in front of you. The entire movement must remain a constant flow, going from the front position to the back position. Each repetition of the movement is dictated by going from front to back.

**Equipment Needed:** In this exercise, two kickboards are needed in order to perform the movement.

9)   Stair Master

**What it is:** This is an exercise that is performed while mostly submerged in the water. It involves grasping onto the stairs with your feet and holding a pool noodle. The exercise requires the body to stabilize in place, which provides a great workout for the core muscles. It also effectively strengthens the arms and back and the hips come into play as well as stabilizers.

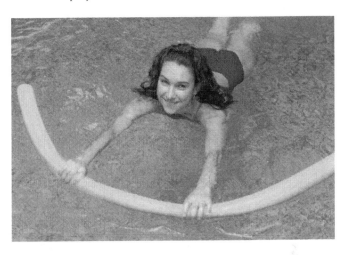

**What to do:** Stick your feet to the ladder of the pool. Hold onto a pool noodle in front of you with both of your hands. Keep a shoulder-width stance and have your arms extended out. Tighten your core to provide stabilization and start pressing the pool noodle towards the bottom of the pool. While performing the movement, make sure to keep the arms straightened until you reach a planking position, as demonstrated in the image above. Hold this position for a total of 30 seconds and return to your starting position. This counts as one repetition.

**Equipment Needed:** As illustrated, only a pool noodle is needed in order to properly perform this exercise.

However, you must be working out in a pool with a ladder attached that you can grip onto with your feet.

10) Knee-to-Chest Crunches

**What it is:** Think of this exercise as a typical abdominal crunch, except for the fact that it is performed in water. The only major difference is that it is often performed like the Roman Chair variation, which requires an almost sitting upright posture before beginning the movement. Regardless, this is a highly effective way to target the core and the abs will get a crazy burn from it, especially with the added resistance caused by the water.

**What to do:** To make this exercise a little easier to execute, many will choose to hold onto the edge of the pool or something else that can keep them fixed in place. Regardless, the movement simply consists of tightening the abs and lifting the knees to the chest in a controlled manner. Once you have returned to the starting position, you will have performed one repetition.

Doing this exercise completely in water with no assistance can be tough. Without any support or a floatation device, the individual will be limited to doing it completely in water – typically at, or around, neck level in height. By doing this exercise out in the open, you will enforce a higher level of concentration on the core, strengthen your stabilizer muscles, and improve your ability to balance in the water.

**Equipment Needed:** No equipment is necessary to perform this particular exercise. A floatation device may be used, but this is rare. There is no need to add resistance or weight to the movement as it provides all the tension that is necessary for the abs to get what they need from the workout.

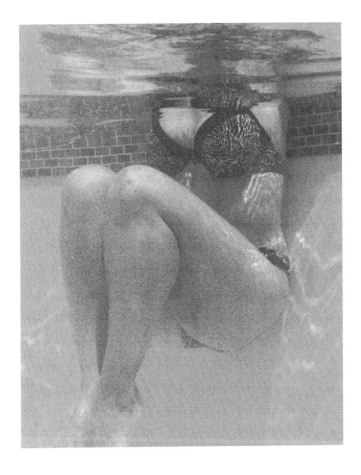

Chapter 6 – Lower Body Workout

A house can only stand strong and firm with proper foundation; the legs can be considered as the foundation for the human body. Not only are they important for their daily functions, but stronger leg muscles also induce better hormone production throughout the entire body. In general, training your legs as well as your upper body will make it easier to improve your overall health and fitness levels.

The lower body is made up of the legs and butt. Some upper body exercises will incorporate the lower half of the body, but typically this is for the purpose of serving as stabilizers. There are a few compound movements, which require multiple muscle groups, as well, but many choose to divide their workout up separately and select exercises to perform that either target the upper or lower parts of the body.

Here are 10 great examples of water aerobics exercises that work to effectively target the lower body, whether it be the calves, thighs (quadriceps and hamstrings) or butt.

1)   Forward Leg Raise

**What it is:** This exercise is a very simple and straightforward movement, which incorporates the leg muscles. It helps to build balance and effectively strengthens stability in the legs. It is often used as an accessory to the more strength-focused exercises, but it can also be effective as an early exercise in your lower body water aerobics workout. In particular, the hamstring muscles require a considerable amount of effort in order to stabilize and execute the movement.

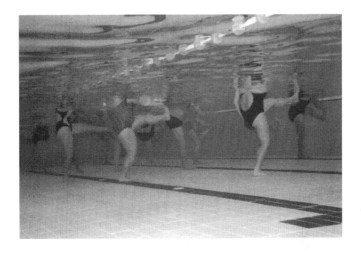

**What to do:** Submerge yourself in water between chest and neck level in height. Keep a strong posture and extend both arms to the side to keep your balance. Stand with your toes pointed to the ground and gradually move one leg up to around waist height, hold in place for up to five seconds, and then return to the starting position. This counts as one repetition. You can alternate between the leg that is used between each repetition, or perform a set of leg raises separately for each side.

**Equipment Needed:** No equipment is necessary for this particular exercise. Ankle weights may be used, but the resistance provided with the water is typically fine for this movement.

2) Backward Leg Raise

**What it is:** This exercise works very similar to the previous one and the only real difference is that the leg is raised backwards instead of frontward. This particular movement may look a little different as the backward leg movement naturally jolts the body forward a bit, but it is essentially the same. Likewise, the targeted muscle will switch a bit as the movement utilizes the quadriceps muscles ahead of the hamstring muscles.

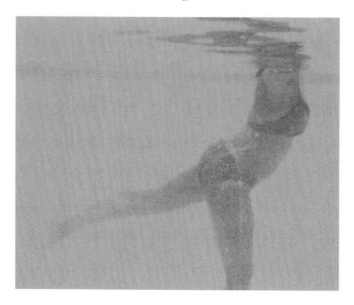

**What to do:** While standing with good posture and feet planted to the ground of the pool, keep your arms extended to the sides to keep yourself balanced. Then, begin the movement by lifting one leg directly behind you as far as possible – without flipping yourself of course!

Your opposing leg will be planted with a bit of a bend in the knee, which may exaggerate a bit as your leg is lifted further back. Once you reach as far back as you are comfortable with, you will then want to hold the position for up to five seconds and then return to the starting position. This counts as one repetition.

**Equipment Needed:** As you can see in the image, pool noodles are being used to perform the exercise. This is not necessary with the frontward leg raises, but it is definitely a good idea when attempting to perform the backward leg raises. It may be a good idea to use a pool noodle when performing this exercise as you will want to keep balance while lifting your leg behind you. Alternatively you may choose to hold on to the side of the pool.

## 3) Side Leg Raise

**What it is:** This exercise is just like the front and back leg raises, except for the fact that the leg is raised to the side. It does not offer anything overly special compared to the other leg raise variations, but it does help with making it easier to switch up the exercises within your leg routine.

**What to do:** With sturdy posture and feet planted firmly on the ground, simply lift and extend one leg out to the side as high as possible. You will not be able to reach a 90 degree angle, but your foot will likely end up just above the opposing leg's knee at the top of the movement. The reverse to the movement is simple enough as you just have to bring the leg back to the starting position. This counts as one repetition.

**Equipment Needed:** No equipment is necessary to perform this exercise.

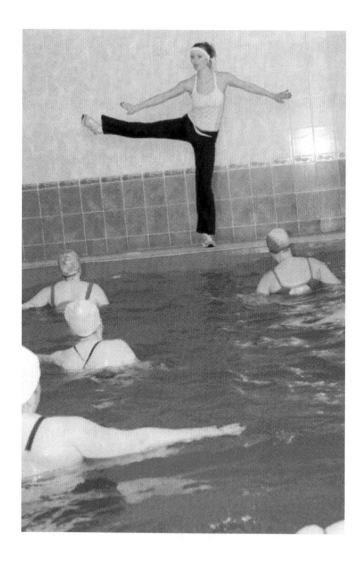

4)   The Bicycle

**What it is:** This exercise operates similar to actual cycling, but it is performed in water! It is a perfect way to get an easy leg workout in and it can be performed by anyone, regardless of their balance and strength.

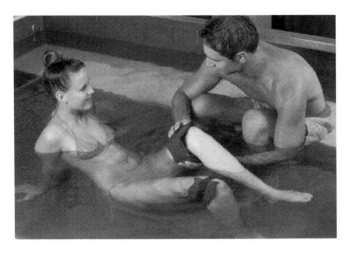

**What to do:** While sitting back on the edge of the pool, hold onto each side of you by grabbing onto the edges with your hands. You will be facing away from the edge of the pool. You will then start the movement by creating a cycling motion with your legs. While doing this, you will want to use a full range of motion and switch between legs after each repetition. You have the option of choosing between performing the movement with the knees directed towards the ceiling, the floor of the pool, or by twisting them to each side.

**Equipment Needed:** No equipment is necessary to perform this exercise. However, equipment such as an ankle weight may be used to increase the difficulty of the movement, or, as in the image, a weight can be attached anywhere on the leg, including above the knee.

5) Kick Backs

**What it is:** This exercise is a fairly straightforward leg-targeted movement that helps to build strength and balance in the lower half of the body. It is done while standing in place and can be performed by just about anyone. It can also be done with or without added resistance, depending on your preferred intensity level and equipment available.

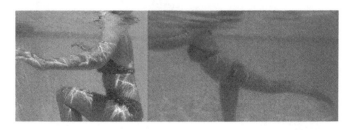

**What to do:** As displayed in the image, you want to stand forward, with your knee slightly bent, and the opposing leg sitting back. This can be done by self-balancing, or by holding onto the edge of the pool. You will begin the movement by bringing your knee in towards your chest and then performing a complete horizontal extension in a backward direction through the force created by your quadriceps and gluteus (butt) muscles. On the retraction part of the movement, your hamstrings and core will get worked due to the resistance. Switch between legs after each repetition and put as much force into your kick back as you want to effectively increase the intensity of the exercise.

**Equipment Needed:** No equipment is necessary to perform this exercise. However, equipment such as an ankle weight may be used to increase the difficulty of the movement.

6)   Mermaid Moment

**What it is:** This exercise takes the motion of swimming like a mermaid and incorporates it into an in-water exercise. It is a great way to target the legs while getting some cardiovascular benefits at the same time.

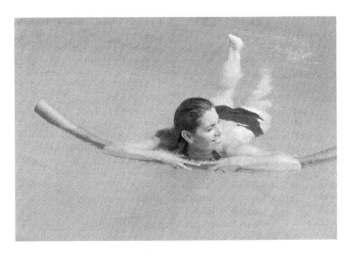

**What to do:** With a pool noodle positioned below your chest and your shoulders above the water, keep your legs extended behind you with a slight bend in the knees and your feet stuck together. You will then begin to extend the legs and continue returning the starting position. By continuously performing this movement, you will be able to push your body forward. This particular exercise does not factor repetitions, but rather is performed at a timed interval, such as for 30 seconds.

7)   Calf Raise

**What it is:** This is a calf-targeted exercise that can produce an incredible burn and works to effectively exhaust the lower leg muscles. It is best near the end of the workout if done with any real level of intensity. It can be thrown into your routine anywhere though, as it serves as a great transitional exercise at a lower intensity level.

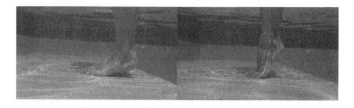

**What to do:** Begin by standing in place. To perform the movement, simply stand on your tippy-toes while extending your calf muscle. Hold at the top of the movement for three to five seconds. For increased difficulty, put a platform at the bottom of the pool and do calf raises on it to increase the range of motion. This makes for a larger stretch of the calf muscle.

**Equipment Needed:** No equipment is necessary for this exercise. However, a platform can be used to allow for a greater range of motion if you wish to increase the intensity of the exercise. Make sure that any type of equipment that is used as a platform is effective for this purpose and will not put the user at risk of slipping off.

8)   Hip Abduction & Adduction

**What it is:** The hip abduction and hip adduction exercises are target the hip abductors and hip adductors, which includes the butt muscles. These are often done with a weighted machine, but can be done in water as well due to the added resistance that the water creates.

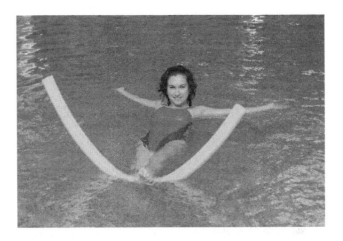

**What to do:** With a pool noodle, place your leg through the noodle with it held in place at around ankle level. With your leg in front of you, begin moving it directly out and to the side. When reaching your full range of motion, reverse the movement and bring it back to the starting position. This counts as one repetition. You can alternate to the other leg after completing one or all of your sets on that side.

**Equipment Needed:** This particular exercise requires a pool noodle to perform as displayed in the picture. Some will choose to do this movement without the noodle, but it is often preferred to use one. As a side note, it is good to stand back on the pool wall if you have any balance issues.

9) Noodle Leg Extensions

**What it is:** This exercise is a simple leg extension, done with a pool noodle for added support and resistance. This movement works to strengthen the upper leg muscles, including the quadriceps, hamstrings, and the butt muscles.

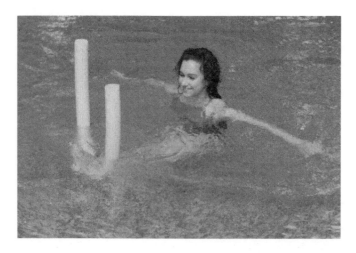

**What to do:** With A pool noodle, place your leg through the noodle with it held in place at around ankle level. With your leg in front of you, begin moving with the pool noodle, lowering your leg to near the bottom of the pool floor and then back to the starting position. This counts as one repetition. You can alternate to the other leg after completing one or all of your sets on that side.

**Equipment Needed:** This particular exercise requires a pool noodle to perform as displayed in the picture. Some will choose to do this movement without the noodle, but it is often preferred to use one. As a side note, it is good to stand back on the pool wall if you have any balance issues.

10) Water Lunge

**What it is:** This exercise is your typical walking lunge, with the only difference being that it is done in a pool. It is used to stretch and strengthen the upper leg and butt muscles. It can be done with or without weights, depending on your fitness level and preferred intensity for this exercise.

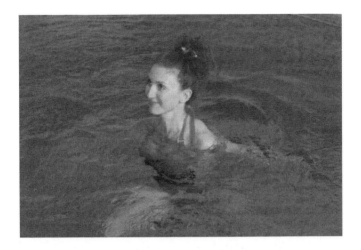

**What to do:** As displayed in the picture, you will want to distance your legs when you move forward and then plant the foot of your front-leading leg down on the bottom of the pool. This will create a bend in the knee, which enforces a stretch of the upper leg and butt muscles. As you step forward with the foot of your supporting leg, you will have returned to your starting position. Instead of counting reps, it is often better to do the water lunge walk for a set distance or a fixed period of time.

**Equipment Needed:** The water lunge can be done without any equipment at all. It can also be done with specialty water weights or any other piece of equipment that will add a bit of resistance to the movement. This will increase the stress on the leg muscles, which ultimately leads to enhanced strength gains for these muscles.

Chapter 7 – Cardio Workout

Getting a full water aerobics workout can only be possible if you include cardio exercises in your routine. This means that you will have to perform cardio exercises, and not just during your warm-up and cool down periods. Although those are the times when cardio is most common.

So, you may not be too sure as to when you should be doing your cardio water aerobics workout. This is understandable as there is no right or wrong time. You can perform your cardio exercises either before or after your body workout, or just schedule an entire day out of your week that is dedicated to cardio.

Regardless of which you choose, it is very important that you know which particular exercises to perform. The reason for this is that there are various cardio exercises, with some being more intense than others, and not all of them are recommended for the entire cardio portion of your workout.

Here are 10 great cardio exercises that you can incorporate into your water aerobics workout:

1) Line Jump

**What it is:** This jumping exercise requires the individual to jump with a cutting in line motion. It is commonly used in training camps for various types of team sports, such as football and basketball. It serves as a great cardiovascular exercise when done at high intensity as you can get a major burn and keep the heart rate up.

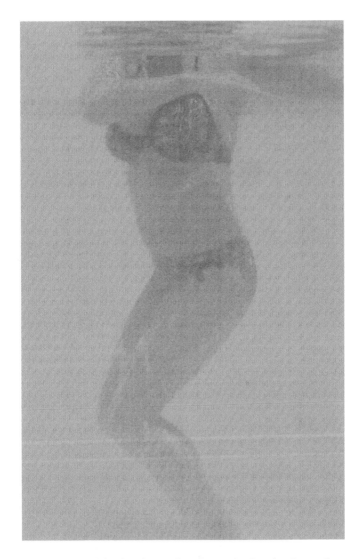

**What to do:** Think of a perfect line, whether horizontal or vertical, in relation to your foot placement. The idea is that you will perform jumps, whether frontward, backward, or to the side, and return to your starting position. During the entire movement, you should be sticking to your imaginary line. While doing this exercise, your legs will likely be kept close together and the movement will feel like a hopping motion.

**Equipment Needed:** No equipment is necessary to perform this particular exercise.

2) Freelance Dancing

**What it is:** This is not an exercise that has been formerly labelled and recommended for cardio purposes, but it is definitely a great way to burn calories and keep your heart rate up. The idea is to get yourself moving and keep moving for a set period of time. You can do this by living out some of your favorite dances, whether it's the Salsa or the "Crank Dat" dance. You don't have to look good doing it, you simply have to keep moving!

**What to do:** Simply hop in the pool and start dancing. Pull a bunch of moves using your legs and arms, move around your hips, etc. Set a period of time to continue dancing in the pool without stopping and choose to modify your intensity levels as you wish.

**Equipment Needed:** No equipment is necessary to perform this particular exercise. Specialty water weights may be used to add intensity to the workout, but this may interfere with the duration at which you can continue dancing for at one time.

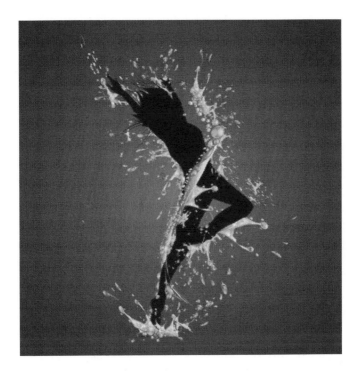

3) Lane Swimming

**What it is:** It's pretty obvious what this particular exercise is, it's simply swimming in a lane pool. While this may not seem like something to suggest for a water aerobics routine, it makes complete sense. Swimming is one of the best forms of cardio to perform and if you are doing water aerobics, you are already in a pool anyway, so there's no real reason not to throw it into your routine.

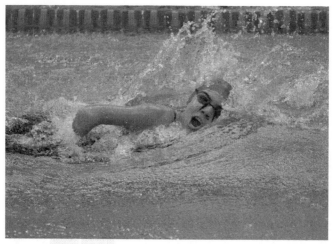

*Photo by* 王伟 *00715*

**What to do:** Hop into the lane pool and start swimming from one end to the other. You can set a certain amount of laps to swim or swim for a certain period of time. You can also play around with the speed at which you swim in the lane pool to set the intensity level for the exercise. For example, you could have a slow steady speed for much of the moment and then perform periodic swimming sprints. The high intensity interval training (HIIT) format is a perfect fit and follows this basic outline.

**Equipment Needed:** No equipment is necessary to perform this particular exercise. As long as you have a lane division within the pool, you will be good to go. If not, you can create your own divider. Further, it is not so important that you have these dividers, but that you perform this exercise as it should be done.

4) Cross Country Ski

**What it is:** This exercise takes from the winter activity of cross country skiing and turns it into a water aerobics exercise. It may seem a little funny to do at first, but once you get the motion down it will prove to be a very easy and effective water aerobics exercise.

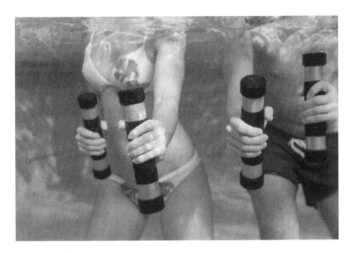

**What to do:** Begin in standing position in the swimming pool with specialty water weights or similar equipment in each of your hands. These will essentially be your skis. You can then begin performing the movement as you would on an actual ski course. The motion may create more of a skipping movement as moving forward in the water will lift you up a bit.

**Equipment Needed:** As mentioned, the specialty water weights or similar equipment that are used in place of skis in your hands are the only piece of equipment that you actually need in order to perform this exercise. Other equipment may be used to add support, resistance, or intensity to the exercise, but it is not necessary.

5) Cycling

**What it is:** It's simply cycling, whether by creating the motion or by actually hopping onto a bicycle. The latter may not seem like it would make sense, but believe it or not, many have actually put an upright exercise bicycle into the pool and used it to perform cycling exercises.

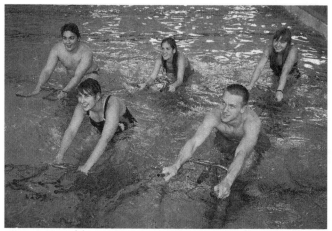

*Photo by http://www.royan.com.au*

**What to do:** As weird as it sounds, throw an exercise book into the pool with the water around chest to neck level, hop on, and start cycling. You can increase or decrease the intensity as you see fit. Typically, this exercise is performed on a timed interval. High intensity interval training (HIIT) format can be used to structure a routine for your cycling exercise.

**Equipment Needed:** An exercise bike is needed to perform this exercise.

6)    Aquatic Zumba

**What it is:** While Zumba has become the most popular craze in the women's fitness industry, aquatic Zumba has followed close behind. Everyone is looking for something to spice up their water aerobics workout and crossing it with Zumba dance classes appears to be the absolute best choice. However, aquatic Zumba is most enjoyed when conducted within a water aerobics class.

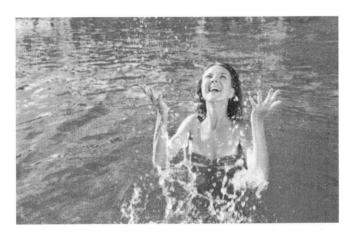

**What to do:** Zumba is a very popular form of aerobic exercise and includes many different movements. As a result, it is impossible to simply explain how to perform Zumba in a pool. However, if you join an aquatic Zumba class, you will be able to perform various movements with no problem at all.

**Equipment Needed:** Whether you need any equipment or not will depend on the plans for the class or what you intend to do within your routine. In most cases, no equipment is necessary to perform this particular exercise.

7)   Aquatic Basketball

**What it is:** Basketball, but played in a swimming pool. This particular form of cardiovascular exercise includes one of the few sports that can be played either alone or in a group while in a pool. It allows for you to set the intensity level at which you are exercising and it is definitely a fun way to get a cardio workout in for the day.

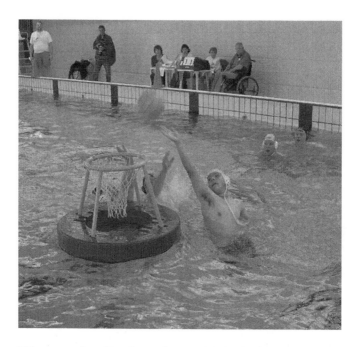

**What to do:** Simply grab a pool basketball and begin shooting it. Try to get the ball into the pool basketball net. As seen in the picture above, the net can actually move in place, which makes sinking the basket even harder. You can move around the pool and play around with shooting form to add some fun to the exercise and there are many different games that you can play if you are working out with at least one other person.

**Equipment Needed:** In the image for this exercise, the individual is using both a floating basketball net and a pool basketball. You will need both a basketball net and basketball that can be used in a swimming pool. However, there are many options for a basketball net. The floating option is good as it prevents the ball from getting out of the pool, but you may prefer the elevated target that comes from setting a short basketball net up on the side of the pool.

8) Captain's Chair With A Twist

**What it is:** This is essentially a movement that is performed with a captain's chair, but the twist comes when the chair is thrown out of the equation and a swimming pool serves as the replacement. This exercise focuses on the abdomen, but serves as a great form of cardio due to the low intensity and consistent stress on the muscle. It is a great addition to your abs workout and serves as an effective transitional exercise between the abdominal and cardio portions of your workout.

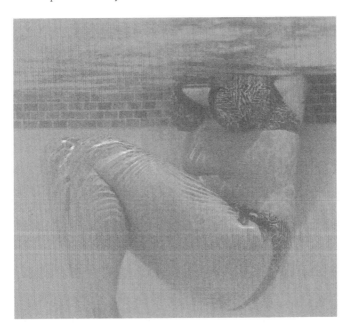

**What to do:** Sit back on the wall of the pool and support yourself by holding onto the pool edge with your hands. Your arms should be rested while doing this. Begin the exercise by bringing your legs together. Lift your knees towards your chest and hold into place. From here, the movement begins by turning your legs while controlling your core and twisting from side to side. You can perform the exercise with a set amount of repetitions, by a fixed period of time, or simply based on the amount of burn that it creates.

**Equipment Needed:** No equipment is necessary to perform this particular exercise.

9) Waist Trimmer

**What it is:** Similar to the exercise before, this movement targets the abdominal muscles. The major difference comes from the difference in leg positioning, with this particular exercise demanding a higher level of intensity. The major difference can be compared by the difference noticed between performing knee raises and crunches on the captain's chair.

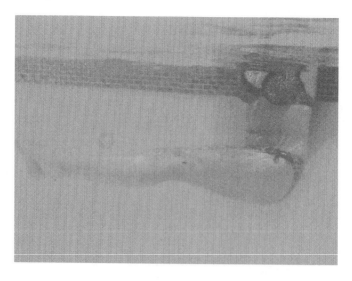

**What to do:** You can position yourself the same as in the previous exercise or use your elbows to support yourself as displayed in the picture for this exercise. This is up to you according to which particular position makes you feel the most comfortable and balanced. Start by kicking your legs up and keeping them together. Bring them as high to chest level as possible. Then, begin moving your legs from side to side while keeping your legs straight. This exercise can be performed by counting the amount of repetitions or by performing the movement for a fixed period of time.

**Equipment Needed:** No equipment is necessary to perform this particular exercise.

10) Aquatic Kickboxing

**What it is:** This one is about as unconventional as it gets. Its kickboxing, like you would do in practice, but it's done in water. The premise of this particular water aerobics exercise is that it is fun and constantly engaging the individual to move around. It may not be as beautiful, or as painful, as it would be in an actual class, but it is definitely a fun way to get your cardio in while working out in the pool.

**What to do:** Simply hop in the pool and begin kickboxing practice. If you do not know the common movements, then you could watch some basic kickboxing training videos before starting the workout. Get your arms and legs going and don't stop until the clock runs out. Rest in intervals to keep yourself going for a long period of time or just use it to fill a few minutes of your cardio routine.

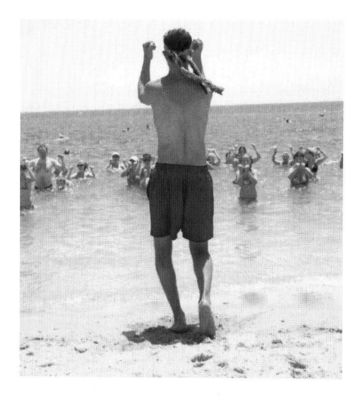

**Equipment Needed:** No equipment is necessary to perform this particular exercise. However, when training with someone else or with a class, punching gloves, pads, and other pieces of equipment may be incorporated to make it easier to train with each other. In reality, the nature of aquatic kickboxing makes movements limited in efficacy and accuracy, so just playing around with stances, strikes, etc., is usually the best way to go about this particular exercise.

Chapter 8 – Planning Your Workout Routine

## What To Know About Creating A Workout Plan

> **Get Started**
> ✔ Consult your doctor before starting an exercise program, especially if you have other health issues or are over 60.
> ✔ Work with a physical therapist/physiotherapist to develop a specific program that meets your needs. A physiotherapist can ensure you are performing activities safely and that they are right for you.
> ✔ Choose a variety of activities to reduce boredom.
> ✔ Have fun! Choosing activities you like will help you stay with a program.

It is important to know how to go about planning your workout routine. This is especially true if you are planning on working out in the pool on your own instead of with a class. However, there are a few things that can interfere with properly creating your workout plan. This section should give you a bit more insight on what to consider when putting everything together.

*Days of the Week*

The first thing you will want to do is decide which days of the week you will be exercising. When deciding this, you can consider which particular muscle groups (if any) you will be targeting on these workout days. It is up to you how many days you wish to work out per week, but two or more is recommended. For instance, you could have two workout days per week with lower body plus cardio and upper body plus cardio, or you could have three days with lower, upper, and cardio.

You can get even more extreme and have an abs day, a legs day, hit the rest of the upper body, then get a cardio day in too, or even just have high and low intensity days. Either way, it is a good idea to keep at least one day of rest after each workout day. This will allow your body to have high energy and strength levels every time you get back into the pool.

Next, you must look further into which exercises you will put into the workout. This is mainly based on the particular muscle groups that they target. So, you will want to definitely write down that "Monday is lower body training day, Wednesday is upper body training day, and Friday is cardio day," or whatever you decide.

*Timeline of the Workout*

You will want to consider how you input each exercise into your workout plan for the day. For example, if you are doing a full body workout, you may choose to do lower or upper body exercises first. This is completely up to you and you can make some adjustments as you see fit after getting a feel for how the workout works for you.

The main fixed factor in this regard is the requirement for sectioning different types of exercise. For example, your warm ups will always come before your main exercises, and your cool downs will always come after your main exercises. When looking at the specific exercises, you may also want to consider whether you should ramp up to the most intense exercise, or if you should plan it out in a different way.

*Reps and Sets*

The reps and sets for each exercise is what confuse many people. Sadly, it is also the most crucial piece of data as it has the largest effect on the intensity of the workout and how tired you feel when you are done. It also plays into the amount of time that you need to rest for, both after each exercise and after each workout.

There is no rule of thumb for setting the appropriate amount of reps and sets for a water aerobics workout. Instead, you will have to look into specific exercises and see what the suggested reps or sets is for that particular exercise. You will not notice any of this in this particular book, but a search online will easily reveal what the recommended reps and sets are for each particular exercise. The reason that this information is not supplied is because it is VERY suggestive – the appropriate amount of reps and sets can vary drastically by individual.

Further, there are many water aerobics exercises that are not performed with actual reps or sets. Instead, these exercises are performed as time-based movements. For example, lane swimming is suggested as a cardio exercise. This can be done by saying each lap is a repetition. However, setting a certain amount of time for this particular exercise can be more rewarding as you can challenge yourself each time to get the most laps possible and because you have full control over the intensity of the exercise.

*Rest Time*

The last thing that you have to think about is your rest time. You will need to make sure that you are getting enough rest both in between your exercises and in between your workout days. The amount of rest that you will need between each exercise will depend on the intensity of the exercise and how exhausted you feel at the time. Generally, you should be able to transition into the next exercise within 30 to 120 seconds, but you can use your own judgment – make sure you are not taking your time just to be lazy though!

In regards to the rest times between specific workout days, it is simply recommended to follow the rule of at least one day of rest before each workout, which means one day of rest after each workout as well. So, on average you would be looking at three workout days per week at the most, but pushing it to four is usually fine. Again, there is nothing better than your own judgment as you know your own body better than anyone else.

Chapter 9 – Water Aerobics For Physical Rehabilitation

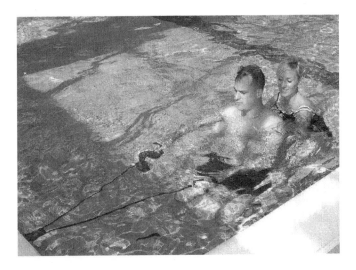

Water aerobics is often suggested for physical rehabilitation purposes. This is because of the fact that water aerobics can be performed by anyone, whether you have a physically restricting medical condition or you are recovering from a physical injury.

An individual undergoing physical rehab will be able to push their limits when needed and decrease the range of motion and exercise intensity if necessary at times as well. In reality, working out in the water can be one of the best ways to strengthen an individual. Especially when rehabbing an injury, working out in the water is perfect as after you have mastered these exercises at varying intensity levels, you will do much better in out-of-water exercises.

A physical therapist does not commonly jump to the suggestion of water aerobics. However, many PT's do have at least a small pool in their building that is used for rehabilitation exercises. This may or may not be enough space, depending on your physical condition.

Regardless, the facts go to show that water aerobics will work wonders for anyone that is rehabbing their injury or trying to strengthen themselves after being diagnosed with a medical condition. Here are some of the reasons why water aerobics may be the right choice:

1. The buoyancy of the water provides support for your weight, which creates a considerable decrease in stress of the joints. This is something that is crucial for many individuals as most out-of-water exercises will create a heavy impact on the joints. Think running and its effects on the joints of the knees.

2. As a result of the lowered impact on the joints, working out becomes much less painful. For someone with arthritis, that experiences frequent joint pain, they will be able to exercise while only feeling a fraction of the stress to the joints, if anything at all. For someone rehabbing an injury, say a fractured bone, they will be able to perform the movements while lowering pain impulses. In this case, the difference sometimes goes unnoticed, but when compared to the severe pain caused by out-of-water exercise with physical injury, the difference is definitely noticeable.

3. So you went and got a sprained ankle, or maybe you tore a ligament? Physical injuries such as these are treated wonderfully by incorporating a water aerobics workout routine into your schedule. The reason for this is simple – the hydrostatic pressure of the water works to lower swelling and also enhances joint positional awareness. The latter is crucial as it leads to better proprioception, which

is affected as a result of these particular types of injuries.

4. Warm water provides comfort and relaxation to the body and its muscles. It also works to make your blood vessels wider and promotes blood flow to the area of the injury. This helps with decreasing the swelling caused by the injury. It is also a great choice for anyone that is looking to decrease the severity of back pain, muscle spasms and various symptoms associated with fibromyalgia.

5. As a result of the combination of everything that working out in water has to offer, you will be able to heal an injury much quicker than you would if you skipped this form of exercise. This is because performing water aerobics workouts will effectively increase blood flow and oxygen to the injured area and because it will help with the removal of potentially harmful toxins from the body as well.

Simply put, water aerobics is one of the few forms of exercise that is both safe and effective for anyone that is recovering from physical injury and for anyone that is dealing with a physically restricting medical problem.

Chapter 10 – Special Conditions

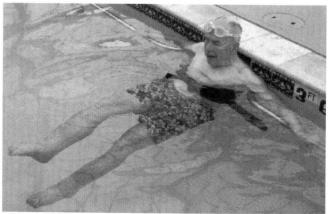

*Photo by Oakley Originals*

Water aerobics is commonly used to treat various medical conditions, such as Parkinson's disease, Multiple Sclerosis and Arthritis. This form of training is very effective at alleviating the painful symptoms that are associated with each of these particular conditions. Aquatic exercise can also effectively help with various restrictive issues with the muscles, joints and bones.

Simply enough, water aerobics serves as a great way to relieve pain and immobility, which is commonly caused by these medical condition examples. However, many do not understand how this is possible and how they should treat aquatic training according to their condition, and this is why many do not go this route when dealing with their medical symptoms.

Since the three listed conditions are very effectively treated with aquatic training, this section will cover all you need to know on using water aerobics exercises if you suffer from any of these conditions.

## Aquatic Training for Parkinson's disease, Multiple Sclerosis and Arthritis

All three of these conditions can affect many aspects of an individual's physical, mental and emotional health. Many of these issues can be remedied by incorporating aquatic training into your fitness regimen. Some examples of changes that may be noticed as a result include an improvement in voice and facial expression functionality, enhanced strength, flexibility, coordination, balance and posture, and an improved range of motion for standard movements of the arms and legs.

There are obvious reasons for all of these changes.

Here are five key points about a water aerobics workout that show how it can be so beneficial when done by an individual suffering from Parkinson's disease, Multiple Sclerosis, or Arthritis:

1.  Being submerged or partially submerged in water creates a greater movement freedom. Basically, think about a simple daily movement of any limb – use lifting your leg up to waist level as an example. Doing this out of water can prove to be very difficult for any individual with Parkinson's, but doing it in water will be noticeably less restrictive. As a result, performing movements in the water creates an improved range of motion for the time-being and makes it easier to perform functional strength exercises.
2.  Being physically active in water creates an almost 'thermogenesis-like' effect as the warm water enhances blood flow and warmth within the body. This thermal effect will ultimately make it easier to lower pain of the muscles, joints and bones, and it

also maximizes one's ability to improve muscular tone as well.

3. The warmth of the water and its natural effects on the human body makes for a soothing and comforting feeling for the body. In return, this makes it a lot easier for an individual to exercise, especially if they are used to feeling discomfort and pain when not in the water.

4. Since there is only a gentle feeling when moving around and exercising in water, muscles are relaxed, able to reach their full length and stiffness is kept to a minimum. This makes it easier and less painful to exercise, which ultimately makes it easier to improve strength, muscular tone, flexibility, coordination, balance, posture, etc., as otherwise, you would be stuck to limited training options.

5. The natural buoyancy caused by being submerged in water makes for a weightlessness feeling for the human body. At the same time, resistance is created while performing movements within the water, even though it feels like the moves are done naturally without any effort. This further contributes towards the list of benefits that have been mentioned. These benefits are made extremely noticeable for individuals that are weaker due to their condition and not exercising because of their symptoms and physical limitations.

*Starting out in water aerobics with Parkinson's disease, Multiple Sclerosis and Arthritis*

If you have not performed water aerobics before, and especially if you have not exercised much recently, you will want to take a few precautions before jumping into the workout.

## Conduct a Sampler Workout

The first thing you will want to do is a sampler workout. This will allow you to get an idea on where you are at right now. It will give you some insight on your current fitness levels and physical ability. This is important as you will want to know what level you can train at and what particular exercises you should perform. After performing your sampler workout, you will know what you need to know in order to be able to go and create your own workout plan.

So, how do you go about creating the sampler workout?

It's pretty simple. Just find a half hour or so to get into the pool and begin trying out all the different water aerobics exercises. You can start out by performing the simple stretches and warm up routines. Then, work into the more demanding exercises. You can start with either upper or lower body exercises and work towards the compound exercises, which incorporate both upper and lower body into the movement. Then, you can test out some cardio exercises and finish off with cool down movements.

After doing this, you will have a general idea on which exercises you can and cannot do. You do not need to push yourself during the sampler workout. You simply need to get an idea for what areas you are limited in and what areas you can work to improve at by beginning to push yourself in later workouts.

## Gathering the Right Equipment

Equipment plays an important role in your water aerobics workout. Without the right pieces of equipment, you will be limited to which movements you are able to perform. There are certain useful exercises that are best done with equipment, such as Noodle Leg Extensions, Mermaid Moment and Centerfold.

If you are performing the water aerobics exercises on your own, then you can always pick up some inexpensive equipment and begin adding to your collection over time. Some of the equipment is only needed for more advanced movements as well, so you can always get these items at a later time when it is actually needed.

Here is a quick list of some pieces of equipment that would be suggested for someone looking to perform water aerobics movements to help with their Parkinson's, Multiple Sclerosis, or Arthritis:

-   Stabilization bar: used to provide balance support while walking in the pool.
-   Pool noodles: used as a floatation device, primarily to create relaxation, and to increase resistance levels during certain exercises.
-   Kick boards: used to improve balance when both sitting and standing and to improve resistance levels during waist exercises.
-   Hand buoys: used to improve resistance levels when performing upper body and core movements and to provide balance support while performing lower body movements.
-   10" diameter balls: used to improve resistance levels for certain waist and arm movements, to perform hand exercises and in games to improve balance.

For anyone looking to perform water aerobics while suffering from any of the three mentioned conditions, it is incredibly important to make sure that you know what you are doing so you get the best results possible.

With that in mind, here are four links that you can use as references to provide you with some more specific information on this subject:

1) http://www.parkinsonswny.com/Aquatic-Handbook.pdf
2) http://www.nationalmssociety.org/living-with-multiple-sclerosis/you-can/exercise-in-water/index.aspx
3) http://sports.yahoo.com/news/water-aerobics-benefits-people-multiple-sclerosis-060400154--highschool.html
4) http://www.arthritis.org/resources/community-programs/aquatics/

**IMPORTANT:** While water aerobics is generally a safe and effective way to train, even for those with physical limitations, there are still some potential risks with this type of exercise. As a result, it is recommended that anyone with a physically-restricting medical condition speaks with their physician or physical therapist prior to beginning a water aerobics workout. This will provide you with the assurance that you need to begin performing these movements.

If you have a physical therapist, then he or she will likely be willing to work with you while performing some of these movements. Even if you plan to do these exercises on your own, you will be able to speak with them for guidance. A physical therapist may also work on a monitoring program with you, so you will be able to track your actual progress and see where you need to improve and make changes to better the results that your workout gives you.

Long story short – do NOT just jump into things and make sure that you consult with your doctor or physical therapist prior to your first workout so you are completely prepared to train.

## Chapter 11 – Now Get In The Pool!!

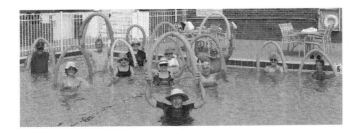

How do you summarize an entire book? It's difficult, especially when so much information has been covered and when some of the most valuable information is in the form of exercise examples. So, let's just look at some of the key points to note about water aerobics:

1) Water aerobics provides a workout platform for everyone, regardless of their age, physical health and current fitness levels. No matter how physically able you are, there will be a range of water aerobics exercises that can cater to you. Whether you want to rehab an injury, improve strength or beat physical symptoms caused by a serious medical problem, water aerobics will have something that is PERFECT for you!

2) Water aerobics is one of the few forms of exercise that effectively offers an insignificant amount of impact on the joints. The decrease in joint impact can vary depending on water height, your weight, and various other factors, but ultimately, you will be taking away a tremendous amount of stress on your joints and ligaments as soon as you decide to take your workout to the pool!

3) Water aerobics is something that you can do alone, with a friend, or with a class. It is completely fun and relaxing – after all, the water

makes it easier to execute many different calorie-burning movements, and you spend the entire workout in a warm pool!

You just can't beat the effectiveness of water aerobics as a primary form of exercise. It is a great choice for conditioning, strengthening, improving endurance and limiting the effects of physical conditions and injuries. Further, working out in the pool is fun and easy, you won't even feel like you're breaking a sweat. Interestingly enough, take the pool full of water away and you would find yourself DRENCHED in sweat.

Long story short, water aerobics is a low impact form of resistance training that can easily help you burn 600 calories or more in only an hour. It is a type of training that allows you to control the intensity and most of the exercises are very fun to do. Also, it is one of those things that you don't really know just how great it is until you actually try it.

For some, this is the ONLY way to exercise. For many, it also happens to be the *BEST* way to work out!

I do hope that you have enjoyed reading this book, and I hope you are ready to get in the water to start burning those calories and toning those muscles. I would be very grateful if you could review this book on Amazon to let others know what you think.

Have a great workout in the pool!!

Printed in Great Britain
by Amazon